THAI
COOKBOOK

70 Easy Recipes for Traditional Food from Thailand

Table of Contents

Introduction

Food is an indispensable part of our every day schedule. Without the addition of solid, nutritious, and scrumptious food, life can truly transform into a test. Cooking is viewed as a difficult task because of the lack of our cooking abilities or exposure to the authentic recipes of different cuisines.

This book is principally about Thai cuisine. Thai food is the public cooking of Thailand. Thai cooking places accentuation on light meals with amazing aromatic segments and a spicy or zesty edge. Thai cooking is about the shuffling of different components to make an amicable completion i.e. like an unpredictable melodic harmony, it must have a smooth surface, yet it does not make a difference what goes on underneath.

In this cookbook, you will come across the history and origin of Thai food as well as the history of traditional Thai dishes. You are going to get a brief information regarding the evolution of Thai cuisine over the years.

There are various health benefits of having Thai food at home, and you will know all of these benefits when you go through the different properties of spices used in Thai foods. You will get over 70 different breakfast, lunch, dinner, and dessert, and authentic recipes that are only eaten by Thai people. You can easily start cooking at home with the detailed instructions present below each recipe.

Preparing your Thai food at home without the need to order food from some restaurant can become very easy, once you start reading this book. So, why wait for more? Let us dive deep into the world of Thai cuisine.

Chapter 1: Introduction to Thai Food

Thailand is the most hailed country in the whole world for its cuisine. From the southern landmass toward the northern locales, the country offers a diverse blend of an irresistibly delightful food.

The south of Thailand is acclaimed for its blazing curries, profound usage of coconut milk, and astonishing fish plans. The northeastern part is striking for its veggie filled plates of blended greens and flavors, grilled meat, sausages, and tenacious rice. Bangkok, the greatest city, attracts Thais from all over the country to make an endless mix of alluring flavors to taste.

From streak cooked sautés to hand beaten servings of blended greens, you can find the variety of mouthwatering flavors. If you value eating, you will be in a paradise with the combination and variety of food in this cuisine.

1.1 History and Origin of Thai Food

Thai food started with the people who emigrated from the southern Chinese regions many years back to the land of Thailand. There was a great Szechwan impact on Thai cooking. In any case, all through the long haul, various things have affected Thai food.

Previously, Buddhist clerics carried an Indian touch to the food, and southern Muslim states influenced the cooking in the south of Thailand. Much later, Thai food was affected by European cooking after contact with Portuguese clergymen and Dutch merchants. During this Time, there was some effect from the Japanese as well.

Thailand is a significant country with a distinct geography, and all through the long haul, this has provoked the improvement of nearby divergences in its style of food varieties.

1.2 History of Traditional Thai Dishes

In the beginning, Thai food was usually eaten while sitting on mats or covers on the floor. These traditions are still found in the more customary and traditional families. Right now, there are four distinct styles of cooking in Traditional Thai food:

- The focal region of Thailand offers food that is somewhere between the north and south. In any case, fragrant Jasmine rice is liked by numerous individuals in the area.

- Southern Thai cooking is the most standard and traditional style for cooking in Thailand since that is the essential tourist territory of the country. In southern cooking, there is significantly more use of coconut milk in various dishes. Coconut replaces Ghee for fricasseeing, and there is a significant usage of fish in majority of their dishes.

- The cooking in northern Thailand is ordinarily milder than in the rest of the country. Firm rice is liked, usually it is kneaded into little balls with the fingers and this is one of the most traditional dishes of Thailand.

- The food in the north east is affected by Laos. The food is astoundingly spiced, and tenacious glutinous rice is the supported staple for north-eastern dishes. Regardless of the point that there are great deals of meat dishes in this section of Thailand, meat was inadequate in these towns, and the highest of protein were shrimp and freshwater fish.

1.3 Evolution of Thai Food over Time

Customarily, while Thai cooking, you do not have to think much as there are a variety of foods available. Thus, arranging food requires heaps of interest and participation, including the family members to cook it all together. The food explains the Thai life and its traditions, customs, and culture. Thai families are gigantic and well-weave. In cooking, Thai family members help each other as a group. In cooking curries, young people assist with light work like nipping off basil leaves, and adults help in pounding chilies and other flavors.

In the current day, making Thai food is much less difficult as each of the ingredients are expeditiously open in general stores, yet there is an examination that it does not have the standard principles of the past.

1.4 Thai Foods According to Nutrition and Dietetics

Thai food is normally adored in the United States, and this food has some amazing nutritional benefits as well. The traditional eating routine of Thailand features striking vegetables, fish, and meats that are given rice or noodles and arranged with flavors like turmeric, galangal, Thai basil, and lemongrass. Food served at Western Thai eateries shares numerous parts of valid Thai cooking, despite the fact that it has some striking contrasts.

Thai menus in America may have greater fragments, more singed nourishments, and plans that are higher in salt and sugar. Following are the curative advantages of Thai food:

- The most generally utilized veggies in Thai dinners are flavorful, like peppers, tomato, cabbage, broccoli, carrots, and onions. These veggies are stacked with fiber, nutrients, minerals, and an assortment of mixtures that add to great absorption and general wellbeing.

- Several of the most well-known Thai ingredients are nutritious, yet there are other sound parts of Thai food. For one, Thai suppers frequently highlight a decent equilibrium of macronutrients like protein, fats, and carbs.

- Eating dinners which to a great extent involve non-bland veggies and furthermore contain protein and fat can assist you with keeping up stable glucose levels for the whole day. This, thusly, prompts supported energy and may help weight reduction.

- Curries, pan-sears, and soups are made with an assortment of vegetables, incorporate a protein source like tofu, lean meat, or fish, and contain coconut milk, nut sauces, or other good fats.

Thai food is known for joining provincial spices and flavors, vegetables, and lean proteins that add both flavor and nourishments to suppers. Nonetheless, some Westernized Thai dishes are pan fried, served in segments, or contain unreasonable measures of added sugar and salt. To pick a solid Thai feast, decide on a dish that are stacked with plant food varieties, contains a protein source, and highlights an assortment of spices and flavors.

1.5 Key Ingredients Used in Thai Food

A large portion of the ingredients found in Thai food are a clear reflection of the environment warm, fertile land and abundant water. Recipes contain fish, unusual products of the soil, a few sorts of noodles and sauces. Rice is the mainstay of most meals. Hot flavoring mixes are utilized to season everything from the day's catch to the easy to make servings of rice or noodles. Following are a portion of the primary ingredients utilized in Thai cooking:

- Cumin: Thai cooks broil fragrant, natural cumin seeds in a dry container to draw out its flavor, and afterward granulate it for use in curry pastes and other zest mixes. Cumin is likewise an essential fixing in many flavor mixes, soups, stews, meat, bean and rice dishes.

- Basil: Basil is utilized both as an enhancing flavor and a topping in Thai cooking. Small bunch of basils are commonly used in soups, curries and sautés.

- Cinnamon: Thai cooks favor Chinese cinnamon, or Cinnamomum cassia, which is better, to some degree spicier, and more uncommon in shading and flavor than Cinnamomum zeylanicum.

- Garlic: Thai cooks use garlic for its health properties, fragrance, and the way that its flavor mixes well with an assortment of different flavors. Garlic is a principle ingredient in the customary Big Four Seasonings Blend, alongside salt, cilantro root, and white peppercorns.

- Cardamom: The fragrant cardamom seedpod is utilized in a couple of Thai dishes of Indian inception, as Mussaman curry. Somewhat lemony, cardamom additionally has a marginally peppery and sweet taste as well as fragrance. Thai cooks frequently consolidate cardamom with other sweet-smelling flavors, similar to cinnamon, nutmeg, and mace.

- Lemongrass: The light, lemony flavor and aroma of lemongrass is an important staple in Thai food. Thai cooks utilize the bulb and base leaves of lemongrass to prepare sauces, soups, pan-sears and curries. It improves meats, poultry, fish, and vegetables, and it is particularly delectable with garlic, chilies and cilantro.

- Turmeric: The robes of Buddhist priests in Thailand are shaded with antiquated yellow color produced using turmeric. Its flavor is sweet, warm, and somewhat peppery. However, it is utilized principally for shading in numerous Thai dishes, including curries, toppings, fish and grain dishes.

- Curry Powders and Pastes: Thais generally mix their own curry powders and pastes by pounding different spices and flavors in a mortar and pestle. Curries are utilized to season coconut milk, serving of mixed greens dressings, noodle sauces, fish and meat dishes, vegetable dishes and soups.

- Chili peppers: Thai food is hot, because of its liberal utilization of new and dried stew peppers. Despite the fact that stew peppers are not local, they are presently fundamental for Thai food.

- Coriander: The strongly fragrant and somewhat interesting kind of coriander seeds is valued in Thai cooking. Thai cooks utilize the root and the leaf of the plant.

- Galangal: A relative of ginger, this light yellow zest has a sharp, lemony, peppery hot taste. It is otherwise called galingale, Java root, or Siamese ginger. Enormous, slim bits of galangal are utilized to season Thai soups, stews and curries; for pastes, it is finely sliced and beat. Ginger might be a replacement for galangal in most Thai plans.

- Mace: It has somewhat nutty, warm taste and found in soups, stuffing, sauces and heated products. It supplements fish, meats, and cheddar, just as certain refreshments.

- Cilantro: Also known as Chinese parsley, Thais utilize this delicate, verdant plant for its unmistakable flavor and natural or amazing fragrance.

- Nutmeg: Thai cooks appreciate the extreme fragrance and sweet, zesty kind of nutmeg in recipes for sweet and appetizing dishes. The chefs utilize a grater to finely powder the nutmeg.

- Cloves: This dim earthy colored, sweet-smelling zest is utilized in the Thai kitchen. Its taste is particular, sharp, and warm or sweet, and you will discover it in both sweet and savory plans.

Thai food will engage any cook who adores the art of seasoning. And while many dishes are very hot, those prepared at home can be adjusted to just the right degree for your own tastes.

Chapter 2: The World of Traditional Thai Breakfast Recipes

Following are some classic traditional Thai breakfast recipes that are rich in healthy nutrients and you can easily make them with the detailed instructions list in each recipe:

2.1 Salapao Recipe

Preparation Time: 30 minutes
Cooking Time: 15 minutes
Serving: 4

Ingredients:

- Sugar, half tablespoon
- Ground pork, half pound
- Soy sauce, one tablespoon
- Finely chopped shallots, one tablespoon
- Chopped garlic, half tablespoon
- Thai pepper powder, half teaspoon

For the dough:
- Vegetable oil, one tablespoon
- Milk, one cup
- Mixed flour, one and a half cup
- Sugar, four tablespoon

Instructions:
1. Take a large bowl.
2. Add the mixed flour and sugar.
3. In a separate bowl, add vegetable oil and the milk.
4. Add the dry ingredients into the wet ingredients.
5. Knead the dough until it turns semi soft.
6. In a pan, add the ground pork.
7. Cook your pork and then add the finely chopped shallots.
8. Cook your pork until the color of the pork changes.
9. Once the color changes, add the soy sauce, sugar, Thai pepper powder and the chopped garlic.
10. Once the pork is done, knead the dough into small round buns.

11. Add the ground pork into the buns and cover the buns all over.
12. Place the buns in the steamer and steam your buns.
13. Steam your buns for ten to fifteen minutes.
14. Your dish is ready to be served.

2.2 Khao Neow Sang Kaya Recipe

Preparation Time: 30 minutes
Cooking Time: 10 minutes
Serving: 4

Ingredients:

- Coconut cream, one cup
- Vanilla extract, one teaspoon
- Eggs, four
- Palm sugar, half cup
- Coconut milk, one cup

Instructions:

1. In a large bowl, add eggs and beat them well.
2. Beat the eggs until it forms a foamy structure.
3. Add the coconut cream and vanilla extract.
4. Beat the mixture and form a fluffy mixture.
5. Add the coconut milk and palm sugar.
6. Mix everything well and form a homogenized mixture.
7. Add the mixture into a greased pan.
8. Add the pan into a steamer.
9. Steam your mixture for ten minutes.
10. Dish out your mixture and cut into pieces.
11. Your dish is ready to be served.

2.3 Khanum Pang (Thai Waffles) Recipe

Preparation Time: 30 minutes
Cooking Time: 10 minutes
Serving: 4

Ingredients:

- Rice flour, one cup
- Eggs, two
- Chopped fresh cilantro, half cup
- Coconut milk, one cup
- Salt to taste
- Shredded coconut, half cup
- Cardamom powder, two tablespoon

Instructions:
1. Heat your waffle maker.
2. Always remember you heat your waffle maker till the point that it starts producing steam.
3. Remove the egg whites in a bowl and beat them to the point that they become fluffy.
4. Beat the egg yolks in a separate bowl.
5. Add in the egg yolks in the egg whites and delicately mix them with a spatula.
6. Combine the eggs and the rest of the ingredients.
7. When your waffle maker is heated adequately, pour in the mixture.
8. Close your waffle maker.
9. Let your waffle cook for five to six minutes approximately.
10. When your waffles are done, dish them out.
11. Add on top of the waffles the chopped cilantro leaves.
12. Your dish is ready to be served.

2.4 Khanom Recipe

Preparation Time: 30 minutes
Cooking Time: 25 minutes
Serving: 4

Ingredients:

- Cornstarch, three tablespoon
- Salt, as required
- Fresh chopped chives, two tablespoon
- Full-fat coconut milk, two cups
- Unsweetened shredded coconut, a quarter cup
- Rice flour, two cups
- Sugar, half cup
- White rice (cooked), three tablespoon

- Canola oil, as required

Instructions:

1. In a large bowl add the coconut milk.
2. With the help of an electrical beater, beat the coconut milk for approximately ten minutes.
3. You will see that after ten minutes, the coconut milk would be fluffy.
4. In a grinder, add the white rice and unsweetened shredded coconut.
5. Grind your ingredients into a fine paste without any granules.
6. Now add this mixture into the beaten coconut milk.
7. Fold your mixture well.
8. Add the rice flour, cornstarch and sugar into the mixture.
9. The mixture will become a little heavier but remember not to beat the mixture, rather fold it so the air spaces are kept intact.
10. Mix all the left ingredients into the coconut milk mixture.
11. In a muffin tray, add your coconut milk mixture.
12. Grease the muffin tray with canola oil.
13. Steam your mixture for approximately ten to fifteen minutes.
14. When your khanom is cooked, dish it out.
15. Your dish is ready to be served.

2.5 Khai Luak (Thai Soft Eggs) Recipe

Preparation Time: 30 minutes
Cooking Time: 10 minutes
Serving: 4

Ingredients:

- Vegetable oil, one and a half tablespoon
- Cooked pork chops, one cup
- Eggs, four
- Sliced scallions, four
- Sliced shallots, two medium sized
- Cooked barley, one cup
- Fresh coriander leaves, half cup
- Fish sauce, one tablespoon
- Lime juice, two tablespoon
- Sliced red chili, one long

Instructions:

1. In a medium bowl, mix together the lime juice, fish sauce, one teaspoon of the chili paste, and the cooked grains.
2. Put the eggs and the excess half teaspoon of chili paste in a little bowl.
3. Beat with a fork to mix everything.
4. In a huge weighty sauté dish, heat half tablespoon of the oil over medium-high warmth.
5. Add the shallots, the white areas of the scallions, and the pork, (if utilizing) and cook, blending infrequently, until the shallots are dim earthy colored and withered.
6. Cook for four more minutes.
7. Add the scallion greens and the leftover half tablespoon of oil and cook briefly.
8. Pour in the egg blend and cook for thirty seconds, at that point turn and mix your eggs.
9. Pour in the mixture of the grain and cook, turning with a spatula, until it is cooked properly.
10. Your dish is ready to be served.

2.6 Khao Rad Gyang (Thai Breakfast Rice and Curry) Recipe

Preparation Time: 30 minutes
Cooking Time: 10 minutes
Serving: 4

Ingredients:

- Thai chilies, two
- Jalapeno, one large
- Sliced green onions, half cup
- White peppercorns, one teaspoon
- Cilantro, one cup
- Fresh ginger, one teaspoon
- Fish sauce, one tablespoon
- Soy sauce, one tablespoon
- Chinese 5 spice, half teaspoon
- Chili garlic sauce, two tablespoon
- Fresh cilantro leaves, half cup
- Thai basil leaves, a quarter cup

- Beef broth, one can
- Minced lemon grass, one teaspoon
- Egg, one large
- Cooked rice, as required

Instructions:
1. Add all the ingredients of the curry into a pan.
2. Add the beef broth and sauces into the mixture.
3. Cook your dish for ten minutes.
4. Add the cooked rice into the mixture once the curry is ready.
5. Mix the rice well and cook it for five minutes.
6. Add the egg into the pan by pushing the rest of the ingredients to a side.
7. Cook the egg and then mix the rest of the ingredients into it.
8. Cook your dish for five more minutes.
9. Add the cilantro into the dish.
10. Mix your rice and then dish it out.
11. Your dish is ready to be served.

2.7 Khao Yum (Thai Breakfast Rice Salad) Recipe

Preparation Time: 10 minutes
Cooking Time: 30 minutes
Serving: 4

Ingredients:

- Water, two tablespoon
- Turmeric powder, one pinch
- Salt to taste
- Garlic cloves, four
- Cooked rice, one cup
- Mix veggies, one cup
- Olive oil

For Thai Dressing:
- Fish sauce, half tablespoon

- Brown sugar, half tablespoon
- Chopped small chili, one
- Water, one tablespoon
- Peanut oil, one teaspoon
- Rice vinegar, half tablespoon
- Sweet chili sauce, half tablespoon

Instructions:
1. Take a large bowl.
2. Add the ingredients for the dressing into the bowl.
3. Mix everything well enough to form a homogeneous mixture.
4. In the next bowl, add the ingredients for the salad.
5. Add the ingredients for the salad into a pan.
6. Cook your ingredients for five to ten minutes.
7. Add the ingredients into a bowl.
8. Add the dressing on top and mix all the ingredients well.
9. Your dish is ready to be served.

2.8 Thai Breakfast Rice and Shrimp Soup Recipe

Preparation Time: 30 minutes
Cooking Time: 10 minutes
Serving: 4

Ingredients:

- White peppercorns, one teaspoon
- Cilantro, one cup
- Shrimps, 150 grams
- Fish sauce, one tablespoon
- Soy sauce, one and a half tablespoon
- Pork stock, three cup
- Jasmine rice, four cups
- Garlic cloves, four

Instructions:

1. Crush the white peppercorns until they turn into powdered form.
2. At that point, add garlic and cilantro and pound until they are crushed.
3. Add portion of this paste to your shrimps and blend well.
4. Sauté the shrimps in a dish with a drop of oil just until it is cooked through.
5. Deglaze the container with some stock and scratch any pieces of spice adhered to the base.
6. Remove from skillet.
7. Bring the stock to a bubble in a pot, add the other portion of the spice paste and stew briefly.
8. Season with fish sauce and soy sauce, at that point taste and add more if you prefer.
9. When prepared to serve, heat the stock to the point of boiling.
10. Add the rice and the shrimp into the stock.
11. Add the soup into a bowl.
12. Garnish it with cilantro leaves.
13. Your dish is ready to be served.

2.9 Thai Styled Traditional Omelet Recipe

Preparation Time: 30 minutes
Cooking Time: 10 minutes
Serving: 4

Ingredients:

- Bean sprouts, one cup
- Fresh coriander leaves, half cup
- Fish sauce, one tablespoon
- Lime juice, two tablespoon
- Sliced red chili, one long
- Green beans, one cup
- Vegetable oil, one and a half tablespoon
- Sliced mushrooms, one cup
- Eggs, eight
- Sliced red capsicum, one large
- Chopped tomatoes, two medium sized

Instructions:

1. Beat the eggs, quarter cup water, lime juice, fish sauce and a large portion of the chili in an enormous container.
2. Heat two teaspoons of oil in a medium non-stick skillet over medium-high warmth.
3. Cook capsicum and mushrooms, mix, for five minutes or until brilliant and delicate.
4. Add the tomatoes.
5. Cook, mixing, for two minutes or until marginally softened.
6. Boil your green beans in water and then drain them.
7. Combine the mushroom blend, sprouts and beans in a bowl.
8. Warm one teaspoon of residual oil in skillet over medium-high heat.
9. Pour quarter of the egg blend into a dish.
10. Cook for thirty seconds or until just set.
11. Slide the omelet onto a plate.
12. Cover your egg to keep it warm.
13. Garnish by sprinkling with coriander and chili.
14. Your dish is ready to be served.

2.10 Thai Breakfast Ginger and Rice Soup Recipe

Preparation Time: 30 minutes
Cooking Time: 10 minutes
Serving: 4

Ingredients:

- White peppercorns, one teaspoon
- Cilantro, one cup
- Ginger paste, two tablespoon
- Fish sauce, one tablespoon
- Soy sauce, one and a half tablespoon
- Pork stock, three cup
- Jasmine rice, four cups
- Garlic cloves, four

Instructions:

1. Crush the white peppercorns until they turn into powdered form.
2. At that point add garlic and cilantro and pound until they are crushed.
3. Add portion of this paste to your ginger paste and blend well.
4. Bring the stock to a bubble in a pot, add the other portion of the spice paste and stew briefly.
5. Season with fish sauce and soy sauce, at that point taste and add more if you prefer.
6. When prepared to serve, heat the stock to the point of boiling.
7. Add the rice and the ginger paste into the stock.
8. Add the soup into a bowl.
9. Garnish it with cilantro leaves.
10. Your dish is ready to be served.

2.11 Spicy Thai Breakfast Noodles Recipe

Preparation Time: 30 minutes
Cooking Time: 10 minutes
Serving: 4

Ingredients:

- Thai chilies, two
- Jalapeno, one large
- Sliced green onions, half cup
- White peppercorns, one teaspoon
- Cilantro, one cup
- Fresh ginger, one teaspoon
- Fish sauce, one tablespoon
- Soy sauce, one tablespoon
- Chinese 5 spice, half teaspoon
- Chili garlic sauce, two tablespoon
- Fresh cilantro leaves, half cup
- Thai basil leaves, a quarter cup
- Beef broth, one can
- Minced lemon grass, one teaspoon
- Egg, one large
- Cooked noodles, as required

Instructions:

1. Add all the ingredients of the sauce into a pan.
2. Add the beef broth and sauces into the mixture.
3. Cook your dish for ten minutes.
4. Add the cooked noodles into the mixture once the sauce is ready.
5. Mix the noodles well and cook it for five minutes.
6. Add the egg into the pan by pushing the rest of the ingredients to a side.
7. Cook the egg and then mix the rest of the ingredients into it.
8. Cook your dish for five more minutes.
9. Add the cilantro into the dish.
10. Mix your noodles and then dish it out.
11. Your dish is ready to be served.

2.12 Thai Fried Eggs Recipe

Preparation Time: 30 minutes
Cooking Time: 10 minutes
Serving: 4

Ingredients:

- Spring onions, four
- Tortilla, as required
- Pepper to taste
- Butter, as required
- Salt to taste
- Baby plum tomatoes, four
- Eggs, four
- Cilantro, half cup

Instructions:

1. Put the butter in a pan.
2. Add the spring onions and chili into the small pan.
3. Cook for a couple of minutes until softened.
4. Whisk the milk and eggs in a bowl.
5. Add the eggs to the pan.
6. Fry your eggs.

7. Add the tomatoes and coriander leaves on top.
8. Once cooked, dish it out.
9. Your dish is ready to be served.

Chapter 3: The World of Traditional Thai Lunch Recipes

Following are some classic traditional Thai lunch recipes that are rich in healthy nutrients and you can easily make them with the detailed instructions list in each recipe:

3.1 Thai Coconut and Noodle Soup Recipe

Preparation Time: 30 minutes
Cooking Time: 10 minutes
Serving: 4

Ingredients:

- Galangal, one can
- Chicken stock, two cups
- Minced garlic, one teaspoon
- Palm sugar, two tablespoon
- Shallot, one
- Kaffir lime leaves, four
- Lime wedges

- Lemon grass, two sticks
- Fish sauce, two tablespoon
- Mushrooms, one cup
- Coconut milk, one cup
- Cilantro, a quarter cup
- Noodles, half pound
- Olive oil, one tablespoon

Instructions:
1. Take a large sauce pan.
2. Add the shallots and olive oil.
3. Cook your shallots and then add the mushrooms.
4. When the mushrooms are cooked then add the galangal, chicken stock, and minced garlic.
5. Add the palm sugar and coconut milk.
6. Cook your ingredients until it starts boiling.
7. Add in the noodles, lemon grass and rest of the ingredients into your soup.
8. Cook your ingredients for ten minutes.
9. When your noodles are cooked dish out your soup.
10. Garnish it with cilantro leaves.
11. Your dish is ready to be served.

3.2 Thai Curry Mud Crab Recipe

Preparation Time: 30 minutes
Cooking Time: 10 minutes
Serving: 4

Ingredients:

- Galangal, one can
- Chicken stock, two cups
- Minced garlic, one teaspoon
- Minced ginger, one teaspoon
- Palm sugar, two tablespoon
- Shallot, one
- Kaffir lime leaves, four

- Lime wedges
- Lemon grass, two sticks
- Fish sauce, two tablespoon
- Mix vegetables, one cup
- Coconut milk, one cup
- Cilantro, a quarter cup
- Crab meat, half pound
- Olive oil, one tablespoon

Instructions:

1. Take a large sauce pan.
2. Add the shallots and olive oil.
3. Cook your shallots and then add the vegetables.
4. When the vegetables are cooked then add the galangal, chicken stock, minced garlic and ginger.
5. Add the palm sugar and coconut milk.
6. Cook your ingredients until it starts boiling.
7. Add in the crab meat, lemon grass and rest of the ingredients into your curry.
8. Cook your ingredients for ten minutes.
9. When your crab meat is cooked dish out your curry.
10. Garnish it with cilantro leaves.
11. Your dish is ready to be served.

3.3 Thai Chicken and Sweet Potato Soup Recipe

Preparation Time: 30 minutes
Cooking Time: 10 minutes
Serving: 4

Ingredients:

- Galangal, one can
- Chicken stock, two cups
- Minced garlic, one teaspoon
- Palm sugar, two tablespoon
- Shallot, one
- Kaffir lime leaves, four

- Lime wedges
- Lemon grass, two sticks
- Fish sauce, two tablespoon
- Sweet potatoes, one cup
- Coconut milk, one cup
- Cilantro, a quarter cup
- Chicken meat, half pound
- Olive oil, one tablespoon

Instructions:
1. Take a large sauce pan.
2. Add the shallots and olive oil.
3. Cook your shallots and then add the chicken meat.
4. When the chicken meat is half cooked, add the galangal, chicken stock, and minced garlic.
5. Add the palm sugar and coconut milk.
6. Cook your ingredients until it starts boiling.
7. Add in the sweet potato, lemon grass and rest of the ingredients into your soup.
8. Cook your ingredients for ten minutes.
9. When your sweet potatoes are cooked dish out your soup.
10. Garnish it with cilantro leaves.
11. Your dish is ready to be served.

3.4 Thai Pork and Peanut Curry Recipe

Preparation Time: 30 minutes
Cooking Time: 10 minutes
Serving: 4

Ingredients:

- Galangal, one can
- Chicken stock, two cups
- Minced garlic, one teaspoon
- Minced ginger, one teaspoon
- Chopped onion, half cup
- Kaffir lime leaves, four

- Minced ginger, half tablespoon
- Lemon grass, two sticks
- Fish sauce, two tablespoon
- Peanuts, one cup
- Coconut milk, one cup
- Cilantro, a quarter cup
- Pork meat, half pound
- Olive oil, one tablespoon

Instructions:

1. Take a large sauce pan.
2. Add the chopped onion and olive oil.
3. Cook your chopped onion and then add the pork meat.
4. When the pork meat is half cooked then add the galangal, chicken stock, minced garlic and ginger.
5. Add the coconut milk.
6. Cook your ingredients until it starts boiling.
7. Add in the peanuts, lemon grass and rest of the ingredients into your curry.
8. Cook your ingredients for ten minutes.
9. When the pork meat is cooked completely, dish out your curry.
10. Garnish it with cilantro leaves.
11. Your dish is ready to be served.

3.5 Thai Beef Stir-Fry Recipe

Preparation Time: 10 minutes
Cooking Time: 20 minutes
Serving: 4

Ingredients:

- Fish sauce, two tablespoon
- Soy sauce, half cup
- Beef pieces, three cups
- Tomatoes, two
- Cilantro, half cup
- Salt and pepper, to taste

- Minced ginger, half tablespoon
- Vegetable oil, two tablespoon
- Thai chili peppers, three
- Toasted nuts, half cup
- Onion, one
- Scallions, half cup
- Minced garlic, one teaspoon

Instructions:
1. In a large sauce pan add the shallots and oil.
2. Cook your shallots and then add the ginger and garlic.
3. Cook your ginger and garlic and then add in the beef pieces.
4. Stir fry your beef pieces well.
5. Add all the spices and the rest of the ingredients into your dish except the toasted nuts.
6. When your beef is cooked then add the toasted nuts.
7. Cook your dish for five minutes.
8. Garnish your dish with cilantro.
9. Your dish is ready to be served.

3.6 Thai Minced Chicken Salad Recipe

Preparation Time: 10 minutes
Cooking Time: 20 minutes
Serving: 4

Ingredients:

- Water, two tablespoon
- Turmeric powder, one pinch
- Salt to taste
- Garlic cloves, four
- Cooked chicken mince, one cup
- Olive oil

For Thai Dressing:
- Fish sauce, half tablespoon
- Brown sugar, half tablespoon

- Chopped small chili, one
- Water, one tablespoon
- Peanut oil, one teaspoon
- Rice vinegar, half tablespoon
- Sweet chili sauce, half tablespoon

Instructions:
1. Take a large bowl.
2. Add the ingredients for the dressing into the bowl.
3. Mix everything well enough to form a consistent mixture.
4. In the next bowl, add the ingredients for the salad.
5. Add the ingredients for the salad into a pan.
6. Cook your ingredients for five to ten minutes.
7. Add the ingredients into a bowl.
8. Add the dressing on top and mix all the ingredients well.
9. Your dish is ready to be served.

3.7 Thai Lemongrass Beef Stew with Noodles Recipe

Preparation Time: 30 minutes
Cooking Time: 10 minutes
Serving: 4

Ingredients:

- Galangal, one can
- Beef stock, two cups
- Minced garlic, one teaspoon
- Palm sugar, two tablespoon
- Shallot, one
- Ginger pieces, a quarter cup
- Beef pieces, half pound
- Kaffir lime leaves, four
- Lemon grass, two sticks
- Fish sauce, two tablespoon
- Mixed vegetables, one cup
- Coconut milk, one cup

- Cilantro, a quarter cup
- Noodles, half pound
- Olive oil, one tablespoon

Instructions:

1. Take a large sauce pan.
2. Add the shallots and olive oil.
3. Cook your shallots and then add the mixed vegetables.
4. When the vegetables are cooked then add the galangal, beef stock, and minced garlic.
5. Add the ginger pieces and coconut milk.
6. Cook your ingredients until it starts boiling.
7. Add in the noodles, lemon grass and rest of the ingredients into your soup.
8. Cook your ingredients for ten minutes.
9. When your noodles are cooked dish out your soup.
10. Garnish it with cilantro leaves.
11. Your dish is ready to be served.

3.8 Thai Butternut Squash Soup Recipe

Preparation Time: 30 minutes
Cooking Time: 10 minutes
Serving: 4

Ingredients:

- Galangal, one can
- vegetables stock, two cups
- Minced garlic, one teaspoon
- Palm sugar, two tablespoon
- Shallot, one
- Ginger pieces, a quarter cup
- Butternut squash, half pound
- Kaffir lime leaves, four
- Lemon grass, two sticks

- Fish sauce, two tablespoon
- Coconut milk, one cup
- Cilantro, a quarter cup
- Noodles, half pound
- Olive oil, one tablespoon

Instructions:
1. Take a large sauce pan.
2. Add the shallots and olive oil.
3. Cook your shallots and then add the butternut squash.
4. When the squash is cooked then add the galangal, vegetable stock, and minced garlic.
5. Add the ginger pieces and coconut milk.
6. Cook your ingredients until it starts boiling.
7. Add in the lemon grass and rest of the ingredients into your soup.
8. Cook your ingredients for ten minutes.
9. Garnish it with cilantro leaves.
10. Your dish is ready to be served.

3.9 Thai Green Chicken Soup Recipe

Preparation Time: 30 minutes
Cooking Time: 10 minutes
Serving: 4

Ingredients:

- Galangal, one can
- Chicken stock, two cups
- Minced garlic, one teaspoon
- Palm sugar, two tablespoon
- Shallot, one
- Kaffir lime leaves, four
- Lime wedges

- Lemon grass, two sticks
- Fish sauce, two tablespoon
- Thai green curry paste, two tablespoon
- Coconut milk, one cup
- Cilantro, a quarter cup
- Chicken meat, half pound
- Olive oil, one tablespoon

Instructions:

1. Take a large sauce pan.
2. Add the shallots and olive oil.
3. Cook your shallots and then add the chicken meat.
4. When the chicken meat is half cooked, add the galangal, green curry paste, chicken stock, and minced garlic.
5. Add the palm sugar and coconut milk.
6. Cook your ingredients until it starts boiling.
7. Add in the lemon grass and rest of the ingredients into your soup.
8. Cook your ingredients for ten minutes.
9. When your chicken meat is cooked completely, dish out your soup.
10. Garnish it with cilantro leaves.
11. Your dish is ready to be served.

3.10 Thai Baked Chicken and Rice Recipe

Preparation Time: 30 minutes
Cooking Time: 25 minutes
Serving: 4

Ingredients:

- Minced ginger, two tablespoon
- Cilantro, half cup
- Olive oil, two tablespoon
- Chopped tomatoes, one cup
- Powdered cumin, one tablespoon
- Salt, to taste
- Black pepper, to taste

- Turmeric powder, one teaspoon
- Fresh Thai herbs, two tablespoon
- Onion, one cup
- Smoked paprika, half teaspoon
- Whole chicken, one pound
- Minced garlic, two tablespoon
- Cooked jasmine rice, as required

Instructions:

1. Take a pan.
2. Add in the oil and onions.
3. Cook the onions until they become soft and fragrant.
4. Add in the chopped garlic and ginger.
5. Cook the mixture and add the tomatoes into it.
6. Add the spices.
7. When the tomatoes are done, add the chicken into it.
8. Mix the chicken so that the tomatoes and spices are coated all over the chicken.
9. Place the chicken on a baking tray and cover your chicken with aluminum foil.
10. Place fresh Thai herbs in the chicken.
11. Bake your chicken for fifteen to twenty minutes.
12. When your chicken is done, dish it out.
13. Sprinkle the cilantro on top of the chicken.
14. Cut your chicken into pieces and place it on the jasmine rice.
15. Your dish is ready to be served.

3.11 Thai Pork Belly with Basil and Tofu Recipe

Preparation Time: 30 minutes
Cooking Time: 10 minutes
Serving: 4

Ingredients:

- Thai chilies, two
- Jalapeno, one large
- Sliced green onions, half cup
- Pork belly pieces, two cups

- Tofu cubes, two cups
- White peppercorns, one teaspoon
- Cilantro, one cup
- Fresh ginger, one teaspoon
- Fish sauce, one tablespoon
- Soy sauce, one tablespoon
- Chinese 5 spice, half teaspoon
- Chili garlic sauce, two tablespoon
- Fresh cilantro leaves, half cup
- Thai basil leaves, a quarter cup
- Chicken broth, one can
- Minced lemon grass, one teaspoon

Instructions:
1. Add all the ingredients of the sauce into a pan.
2. Add the chicken broth and sauces into the mixture.
3. Cook your dish for ten minutes.
4. Add the pork belly pieces and tofu pieces into the mixture once the sauce is ready.
5. Mix the ingredients well and cook it for five minutes.
6. Add the basil leaves and then mix the rest of the ingredients into it.
7. Cook your dish for five more minutes.
8. Add the cilantro into the dish.
9. Your dish is ready to be served.

3.12 Thai Red Meatball Curry Recipe

Preparation Time: 30 minutes
Cooking Time: 10 minutes
Serving: 4

Ingredients:

- Galangal, one can
- Chicken stock, two cups
- Minced garlic, one teaspoon
- Palm sugar, two tablespoon
- Shallot, one

- Kaffir lime leaves, four
- Lime wedges
- Lemon grass, two sticks
- Fish sauce, two tablespoon
- Thai red curry paste, two tablespoon
- Coconut milk, one cup
- Cilantro, a quarter cup
- Frozen meatballs, half pound
- Olive oil, one tablespoon

Instructions:
1. Take a large sauce pan.
2. Add the shallots and olive oil.
3. Cook your shallots and then add the meatballs.
4. When the meatballs are half cooked, add the galangal, red curry paste, chicken stock, and minced garlic.
5. Add the palm sugar and coconut milk.
6. Cook your ingredients until it starts boiling.
7. Add in the lemon grass and rest of the ingredients into the curry.
8. Cook your ingredients for ten minutes.
9. When your curry is cooked dish it out.
10. Garnish it with cilantro leaves.
11. Your dish is ready to be served.

3.13 Thai Sesame Chicken Salad Recipe

Preparation Time: 10 minutes
Cooking Time: 20 minutes
Serving: 4

Ingredients:

- White sesame seeds, half cup
- Black sesame seeds, half cup
- Salt to taste
- Garlic cloves, four
- Cooked chicken meat, one cup

- Olive oil

For Thai Dressing:
- Fish sauce, half tablespoon
- Brown sugar, half tablespoon
- Chopped small chili, one
- Water, one tablespoon
- Peanut oil, one teaspoon
- Rice vinegar, half tablespoon
- Sweet chili sauce, half tablespoon

Instructions:
1. Take a large bowl.
2. Add the ingredients for the dressing into the bowl.
3. Mix everything well enough to form a smooth mixture.
4. In the next bowl, add the ingredients for the salad.
5. Add the ingredients for the salad into a bowl.
6. Add the dressing on top and mix all the ingredients well.
7. Your dish is ready to be served.

3.14 Spicy Thai Prawn Noodles Recipe

Preparation Time: 30 minutes
Cooking Time: 10 minutes
Serving: 4

Ingredients:

- Thai chilies, two
- Jalapeno, one large
- Sliced green onions, half cup
- White peppercorns, one teaspoon
- Cilantro, one cup
- Fresh ginger, one teaspoon
- Fish sauce, one tablespoon
- Soy sauce, one tablespoon
- Chinese 5 spice, half teaspoon
- Chili garlic sauce, two tablespoon

- Fresh cilantro leaves, half cup
- Prawns, two cups
- Fish broth, one can
- Minced lemon grass, one teaspoon
- Cooked noodles, as required

Instructions:

1. Add all the ingredients of the sauce into a pan.
2. Add the fish broth and sauces into the mixture.
3. Cook your dish for ten minutes.
4. Add the cooked noodles into the mixture once the sauce is ready.
5. Mix the noodles well and cook it for five minutes.
6. Add the prawns into the pan by pushing the rest of the ingredients to a side.
7. Cook the prawns and then mix the rest of the ingredients into it.
8. Cook your dish for five more minutes.
9. Add the cilantro into the dish.
10. Mix your noodles and then dish it out.
11. Your dish is ready to be served.

3.15 Thai Red Salmon Curry Recipe

Preparation Time: 30 minutes
Cooking Time: 10 minutes
Serving: 4

Ingredients:

- Galangal, one can
- Fish stock, two cups
- Minced garlic, one teaspoon
- Shallot, one
- Kaffir lime leaves, four
- Lemon grass, two sticks
- Fish sauce, two tablespoon
- Thai red curry paste, two tablespoon
- Cilantro, a quarter cup

- Salmon meat, half pound
- Olive oil, one tablespoon

Instructions:
1. Take a large sauce pan.
2. Add the shallots and olive oil.
3. Cook your shallots and then add the salmon meat.
4. When the salmon meat is half cooked, add the galangal, red curry paste, fish stock, and minced garlic.
5. Cook your ingredients until it starts boiling.
6. Add in the lemon grass and rest of the ingredients into the curry.
7. Cook your ingredients for ten minutes.
8. When your curry is cooked dish it out.
9. Garnish it with cilantro leaves.
10. Your dish is ready to be served.

Chapter 4: The World of Traditional Thai Dinner Recipes

Following are some classic traditional Thai dinner recipes that are rich in healthy nutrients and you can easily make them with the detailed instructions list in each recipe:

4.1 Thai Peanut Chicken and Noodles Recipe

Preparation Time: 30 minutes
Cooking Time: 10 minutes
Serving: 4

Ingredients:

- Galangal, one can
- Chicken stock, two cups
- Minced garlic, one teaspoon
- Minced ginger, one teaspoon
- Chopped onion, half cup
- Noodles, two cups
- Minced ginger, half tablespoon
- Lemon grass, two sticks
- Fish sauce, two tablespoon
- Peanuts, one cup
- Coconut milk, one cup
- Cilantro, a quarter cup
- Chicken meat, half pound
- Olive oil, one tablespoon

Instructions:

1. Take a large sauce pan.
2. Add the chopped onion and olive oil.
3. Cook your chopped onion and then add the chicken meat.
4. When the chicken meat is half cooked then add the galangal, chicken stock, minced garlic and ginger.
5. Add the coconut milk.
6. Cook your ingredients until it starts boiling.
7. Add in the noodles, peanuts, lemon grass and rest of the ingredients into your curry.
8. Cook your ingredients for ten minutes.
9. Garnish it with cilantro leaves.
10. Your dish is ready to be served.

4.2 Thai Red Curry Chicken and Vegetable Recipe

Preparation Time: 30 minutes
Cooking Time: 10 minutes
Serving: 4

Ingredients:

- Galangal, one can
- Chicken stock, two cups
- Minced garlic, one teaspoon
- Shallot, one
- Mix vegetables, one cup
- Lemon grass, two sticks
- Fish sauce, two tablespoon
- Thai red curry paste, two tablespoon
- Cilantro, a quarter cup
- Chicken meat, half pound
- Olive oil, one tablespoon

Instructions:
1. Take a large sauce pan.
2. Add the shallots and olive oil.
3. Cook your shallots and then add the chicken meat and vegetables.
4. When the chicken meat is half cooked, add the galangal, red curry paste, chicken stock, and minced garlic.
5. Cook your ingredients until it starts boiling.
6. Add in the lemon grass and rest of the ingredients into the dish.
7. Cook your ingredients for ten minutes.
8. Garnish it with cilantro leaves.
9. Your dish is ready to be served.

4.3 Thai Noodles with Spicy Peanut Sauce Recipe

Preparation Time: 30 minutes
Cooking Time: 10 minutes

Ingredients:

- Mixed vegetables, two cups
- Minced garlic, one teaspoon
- Minced ginger, one teaspoon
- Chopped onion, half cup
- Noodles, two cups
- Minced ginger, half tablespoon
- Lemon grass, two sticks
- Fish sauce, two tablespoon
- Spicy peanut sauce, one cup
- Coconut milk, one cup
- Cilantro, a quarter cup
- Olive oil, one tablespoon

Instructions:
1. Take a large sauce pan.
2. Add the chopped onion and olive oil.
3. Cook your chopped onion and then add the vegetables.
4. Add the coconut milk.
5. Cook your ingredients until it starts boiling.
6. Add in the noodles, spicy peanut sauce and the rest of the ingredients.
7. Cook your ingredients for ten minutes.
8. Garnish it with cilantro leaves.
9. Your dish is ready to be served.

4.4 Thai Coconut and Beef Curry Recipe

Preparation Time: 30 minutes
Cooking Time: 10 minutes
Serving: 4

Ingredients:

- Galangal, one can

- Beef stock, two cups
- Minced garlic, one teaspoon
- Crushed ginger, one teaspoon
- Chopped onion, half cup
- Minced ginger, half tablespoon
- Lemon grass, two sticks
- Fish sauce, two tablespoon
- Shredded coconut, one cup
- Coconut milk, one cup
- Cilantro, a quarter cup
- Beef meat, half pound
- Olive oil, one tablespoon

Instructions:

1. Take a large sauce pan.
2. Add the chopped onion and olive oil.
3. Cook your chopped onion and then add the beef meat.
4. When the beef meat is half cooked then add the galangal, beef stock, minced garlic and ginger.
5. Add the coconut milk.
6. Cook your ingredients until it starts boiling.
7. Add in the shredded coconut, lemon grass and rest of the ingredients into your curry.
8. Cook your ingredients for ten minutes.
9. When your beef meat is cooked completely dish out your curry.
10. Garnish it with cilantro leaves.
11. Your dish is ready to be served.

4.5 Thai Coconut and Beef Salad Recipe

Preparation Time: 10 minutes
Cooking Time: 20 minutes
Serving: 4

Ingredients:

- Water, two tablespoon

- Shredded coconut, half cup
- Salt to taste
- Garlic cloves, four
- Cooked beef strips, one cup
- Olive oil

For Thai Dressing:
- Fish sauce, half tablespoon
- Brown sugar, half tablespoon
- Chopped small chili, one
- Water, one tablespoon
- Peanut oil, one teaspoon
- Rice vinegar, half tablespoon
- Sweet chili sauce, half tablespoon

Instructions:
1. Take a large bowl.
2. Add the ingredients for the dressing into the bowl.
3. Mix everything well enough to form a consistent mixture.
4. In the next bowl, add the ingredients for the salad.
5. Add the ingredients for the salad into a bowl and mix properly.
6. Add the dressing on top and mix all the ingredients well.
7. Your dish is ready to be served.

4.6 Thai Green Chicken Thighs Recipe

Preparation Time: 10 minutes
Cooking Time: 40 minutes
Serving: 2

Ingredients:

- Chicken broth, one cup
- Thai green curry paste, one teaspoon
- Onion, one cup
- Lemon juice, half cup
- Chicken thighs, half pound
- Thai spices, half tablespoon

- Water, one cup
- Minced garlic, two tablespoon
- Minced ginger, two tablespoon
- Cilantro, half cup
- Olive oil, two tablespoon
- Chopped tomatoes, one cup

Instructions:

1. Take a pan.
2. Add in the oil and onions.
3. Cook the onions until they become soft and fragrant.
4. Add in the chopped garlic and ginger.
5. Cook the mixture and add the tomatoes into it.
6. Add the spices and chicken thighs.
7. Add in the broth.
8. Mix the ingredients carefully and cover your pan.
9. Add cilantro on top.
10. Your dish is ready to be served.

4.7 Thai Basil Pork Stir-Fry Recipe

Preparation Time: 10 minutes
Cooking Time: 20 minutes
Serving: 4

Ingredients:

- Fish sauce, two tablespoon
- Soy sauce, half cup
- Pork pieces, three cups
- Tomatoes, two
- Cilantro, half cup
- Salt and pepper, to taste
- Minced ginger, half tablespoon
- Vegetable oil, two tablespoon
- Thai chili peppers, three
- Basil leaves, half cup

- Onion, one
- Minced garlic, one teaspoon

Instructions:

1. In a large sauce pan, add the onions and oil.
2. Cook your onions and then add the ginger and garlic.
3. Cook your ginger and garlic and then add in the pork pieces.
4. Stir fry your pork pieces well.
5. Add all the spices and the rest of the ingredients into your dish except the basil leaves.
6. When your pork is cooked then add the basil leaves.
7. Cook your dish for five minutes.
8. Garnish your dish with cilantro.
9. Your dish is ready to be served.

4.8 Thai Green Chicken Curry with Vegetables Recipe

Preparation Time: 30 minutes
Cooking Time: 10 minutes
Serving: 4

Ingredients:

- Galangal, one can
- Chicken stock, two cups
- Minced garlic, one teaspoon
- Shallot, one
- Kaffir lime leaves, four
- Lime wedges
- Lemon grass, two sticks
- Fish sauce, two tablespoon
- Thai green curry paste, two tablespoon
- Mixed vegetables, one cup
- Cilantro, a quarter cup
- Chicken pieces, half pound
- Olive oil, one tablespoon

Instructions:

1. Take a large sauce pan.
2. Add the shallots and olive oil.
3. Cook your shallots and then add the chicken pieces and vegetables.
4. When the chicken pieces are half cooked, add the galangal, green curry paste, chicken stock, and minced garlic.
5. Cook your ingredients until it starts boiling.
6. Add in the lemon grass and rest of the ingredients into your soup.
7. Cook your ingredients for ten minutes.
8. When your chicken pieces are cooked completely dish out your soup.
9. Garnish it with cilantro leaves.
10. Your dish is ready to be served.

4.9 Thai Mussels in Basil Coconut Sauce Recipe

Preparation Time: 30 minutes
Cooking Time: 10 minutes
Serving: 4

Ingredients:

- Galangal, one can
- Fish stock, two cups
- Minced garlic, one teaspoon
- Minced ginger, one teaspoon
- Chopped onion, half cup
- Crushed ginger, half tablespoon
- Basil leaves, a quarter cup
- Fish sauce, two tablespoon
- Shredded coconut, one cup
- Coconut milk, one cup
- Cilantro, a quarter cup
- Mussels, half pound
- Olive oil, one tablespoon

Instructions:

1. Take a large sauce pan.
2. Add the chopped onion and olive oil.
3. Cook your chopped onion and then add the mussels.
4. When the mussels are half cooked then add the galangal, fish stock, minced garlic and ginger.
5. Add the coconut milk.
6. Cook your ingredients until it starts boiling.
7. Add in the shredded coconut, basil leaves and rest of the ingredients into your curry.
8. Cook your ingredients for ten minutes.
9. Garnish it with cilantro leaves.
10. Your dish is ready to be served.

4.10 Thai Pumpkin and Sweet Potato Curry Recipe

Preparation Time: 30 minutes
Cooking Time: 10 minutes
Serving: 4

Ingredients:

- Galangal, one can
- Chicken stock, two cups
- Chopped garlic, one teaspoon
- Palm sugar, two tablespoon
- Shallot, one
- Lemon grass, two sticks
- Fish sauce, two tablespoon
- Sweet potatoes, one cup
- Coconut milk, one cup
- Cilantro, a quarter cup
- Pumpkin pieces, two cups
- Olive oil, one tablespoon

Instructions:

1. Take a large sauce pan.
2. Add the shallots and olive oil.
3. Cook your shallots.
4. When the pumpkin and sweet potatoes is half cooked, add the galangal, chicken stock, and minced garlic.
5. Cook your ingredients until it starts boiling.
6. Add in the lemon grass and rest of the ingredients into your curry.
7. Cook your ingredients for ten minutes.
8. Garnish it with cilantro leaves.
9. Your dish is ready to be served.

4.11 Thai Tofu Fried Rice Recipe

Preparation Time: 30 minutes
Cooking Time: 10 minutes
Serving: 4

Ingredients:

- Tofu cubes, one cup
- Jalapeno, one large
- Sliced green onions, half cup
- White peppercorns, one teaspoon
- Cilantro, one cup
- Fresh ginger, one teaspoon
- Fish sauce, one tablespoon
- Soy sauce, one tablespoon
- Chinese 5 spice, half teaspoon
- Chili garlic sauce, two tablespoon
- Fresh cilantro leaves, half cup
- Thai basil leaves, a quarter cup
- Vegetable broth, one can
- Minced lemon grass, one teaspoon
- Cooked rice, as required

Instructions:

1. Add all the ingredients of the curry into a pan.
2. Add the vegetable broth and sauces into the mixture.
3. Cook your dish for ten minutes.
4. Add the cooked rice into the mixture once the curry is ready.
5. Mix the rice well and cook it for five minutes.
6. Add the tofu pieces into the pan by pushing the rest of the ingredients to a side.
7. Cook the tofu pieces and then mix the rest of the ingredients into it.
8. Cook your dish for five more minutes.
9. Add the cilantro into the dish.
10. Mix your rice and then dish it out.
11. Your dish is ready to be served.

4.12 Thai Chicken Pad Thai Recipe

Preparation Time: 30 minutes
Cooking Time: 10 minutes
Serving: 4

Ingredients:

- Mixed vegetables, two cups
- Sliced green onions, half cup
- White peppercorns, one teaspoon
- Cilantro, one cup
- Fresh ginger, one teaspoon
- Fish sauce, one tablespoon
- Soy sauce, one tablespoon
- Chinese 5 spice, half teaspoon
- Chili garlic sauce, two tablespoon
- Fresh cilantro leaves, half cup
- Thai basil leaves, a quarter cup
- Chicken broth, one can
- Chicken pieces, half pound
- Cooked noodles, as required

Instructions:

1. Add all the ingredients of the sauce into a pan.
2. Add the chicken pieces, vegetables, chicken broth and sauces into the mixture.
3. Cook your dish for ten minutes.
4. Add the cooked noodles into the mixture once the sauce is ready.
5. Mix the noodles well and cook it for five minutes.
6. Add the cilantro into the dish.
7. Mix your noodles and then dish it out.
8. Your dish is ready to be served.

4.13 Thai Sour and Spicy Soup Recipe

Preparation Time: 30 minutes
Cooking Time: 10 minutes
Serving: 4

Ingredients:

- Galangal, one can
- Vegetables stock, two cups
- Minced garlic, one teaspoon
- Palm sugar, two tablespoon
- Shallot, one
- Sweet and sour sauce, half cup
- Ginger pieces, a quarter cup
- Lemon grass, two sticks
- Fish sauce, two tablespoon
- Mixed vegetables, one cup
- Coconut milk, one cup
- Cilantro, a quarter cup
- Olive oil, one tablespoon

Instructions:
1. Take a large sauce pan.
2. Add the shallots and olive oil.
3. Cook your shallots and then add the mixed vegetables.
4. When the vegetables are cooked then add the galangal, vegetable stock, and minced garlic.

5. Add the ginger pieces and coconut milk.
6. Cook your ingredients until it starts boiling.
7. Add in the sweet and sour sauce, lemon grass and rest of the ingredients into your soup.
8. Cook your ingredients for ten minutes.
9. Garnish it with cilantro leaves.
10. Your dish is ready to be served.

4.14 Thai Pumpkin and Coconut Curry Recipe

Preparation Time: 30 minutes
Cooking Time: 10 minutes
Serving: 4

Ingredients:

- Galangal, one can
- Vegetable stock, two cups
- Minced garlic, one teaspoon
- Minced ginger, one teaspoon
- Chopped onion, half cup
- Minced ginger, half tablespoon
- Lemon grass, two sticks
- Fish sauce, two tablespoon
- Shredded coconut, one cup
- Coconut milk, one cup
- Cilantro, a quarter cup
- Pumpkin pieces, half pound
- Olive oil, one tablespoon

Instructions:
1. Take a large sauce pan.
2. Add the chopped onion and olive oil.
3. Cook your chopped onion and then add the pumpkin pieces.
4. When the pumpkin pieces are half cooked then add the galangal, vegetable stock, minced garlic and ginger.
5. Add the coconut milk.

6. Add in the shredded coconut, lemon grass and rest of the ingredients into your curry.
7. Cook your ingredients for ten minutes.
8. Garnish it with cilantro leaves.
9. Your dish is ready to be served.

4.15 Thai Grilled Salmon Recipe

Preparation Time: 30 minutes
Cooking Time: 25 minutes
Serving: 4

Ingredients:

- Minced ginger, two tablespoon
- Cilantro, half cup
- Olive oil, two tablespoon
- Chopped tomatoes, one cup
- Powdered cumin, one tablespoon
- Salt, to taste
- Black pepper, to taste
- Turmeric powder, one teaspoon
- Fresh Thai herbs, two tablespoon
- Onion, one cup
- Salmon filet, one pound
- Minced garlic, two tablespoon

Instructions:
1. Take a pan.
2. Add in the oil and onions.
3. Cook the onions until they become soft and fragrant.
4. Add in the chopped garlic and ginger.
5. Cook the mixture and add the tomatoes into it.
6. Add the spices.
7. Mix the salmon so that the tomatoes and spices are coated all over the salmon.
8. Place fresh Thai herbs on the salmon.
9. Grill your salmon for fifteen to twenty minutes.

10. When your salmon is done, dish it out.
11. Sprinkle the cilantro on top of the salmon.
12. Your dish is ready to be served.

4.16 Thai Red Beef Curry Recipe

Preparation Time: 30 minutes
Cooking Time: 10 minutes
Serving: 4

Ingredients:

- Beef stock, two cups
- Crushed garlic, one teaspoon
- Palm sugar, two tablespoon
- Shallot, one
- Kaffir lime leaves, four
- Lemon grass, two sticks
- Fish sauce, two tablespoon
- Thai red curry paste, two tablespoon
- Cilantro, a quarter cup
- Beef, half pound
- Olive oil, one tablespoon

Instructions:

1. Take a large sauce pan.
2. Add the shallots and olive oil.
3. Cook your shallots and then add the beef meat.
4. When the beef is half cooked, add the red curry paste, beef stock, and minced garlic.
5. Cook your ingredients until it starts boiling.
6. Add in the lemon grass and rest of the ingredients into the curry.
7. Cook your ingredients for ten minutes.
8. When your curry is cooked, dish it out.
9. Garnish it with cilantro leaves.

10.   Your dish is ready to be served.

4.17 Thai Coconut Curry Recipe

Preparation Time: 30 minutes
Cooking Time: 10 minutes
Serving: 4

Ingredients:

- Galangal, one can
- Vegetable stock, two cups
- Minced garlic, one teaspoon
- Minced ginger, one teaspoon
- Chopped onion, half cup
- Chopped ginger, half tablespoon
- Lemon grass, two sticks
- Fish sauce, two tablespoon
- Shredded coconut, one cup
- Coconut milk, one cup
- Cilantro, a quarter cup
- Olive oil, one tablespoon

Instructions:

1. Take a large sauce pan.
2. Add the chopped onion and olive oil.
3. Cook your chopped onion.
4. When the onions are cooked then add the galangal, vegetable stock, minced garlic and ginger.
5. Add the coconut milk.
6. Cook your ingredients until it starts boiling.
7. Add in the shredded coconut, lemon grass and rest of the ingredients into your curry.
8. Cook your ingredients for ten minutes.
9. Garnish it with cilantro leaves.
10.   Your dish is ready to be served.

4.18 Thai Pumpkin and Vegetable Soup Recipe

Preparation Time: 30 minutes
Cooking Time: 10 minutes
Serving: 4

Ingredients:

- Vegetables stock, two cups
- Minced garlic, one teaspoon
- Galangal, one can
- Shallot, one
- Pumpkin pieces, one cup
- Ginger pieces, a quarter cup
- Lemon grass, two sticks
- Fish sauce, two tablespoon
- Mixed vegetables, one cup
- Coconut milk, one cup
- Cilantro, a quarter cup
- Olive oil, one tablespoon

Instructions:

1. Take a large sauce pan.
2. Add the shallots and olive oil.
3. Cook your shallots and then add the mixed vegetables.
4. When the vegetables are cooked then add the galangal, vegetable stock, and minced garlic.
5. Add the ginger pieces and coconut milk.
6. Cook your ingredients until it starts boiling.
7. Add in the pumpkin, lemon grass and rest of the ingredients into your soup.
8. Cook your ingredients for ten minutes.
9. Garnish it with cilantro leaves.
10. Your dish is ready to be served.

Chapter 5: The World of Traditional Thai Dessert Recipes

Following are some classic traditional Thai dessert recipes that are rich in healthy nutrients and you can easily make them with the detailed instructions list in each recipe:

5.1 Thai Coconut Pudding Recipe

Preparation Time: 10 minutes
Cooking Time: 30 minutes
Serving: 2

Ingredients:
- Coconut Milk, two cups
- White sugar, half cup
- Salt, one teaspoon
- Eggs, two
- Lemon extract, one teaspoon
- Almond extract, one teaspoon
- All-purpose flour, two cups
- Butter, one cup
- Dry yeast, one cup

Instructions:
1. Take a medium bowl and add the butter in it.
2. Add one cup flour and mix well.
3. Then refrigerate it.
4. Take a large bowl and add yeast into it.
5. Add the sugar, the salt and the milk.
6. Mix them well.
7. Mix the warm milk mixture with the flour and the yeast.
8. Add the lemon extract, eggs and almond extract together.
9. Add the baking soda in the mixture.
10. Simmer it for few minutes.
11. Check the thickness of the pudding.

12.   Serve warm.

5.2 Thai Fruit Salad Recipe

Preparation Time: 10 minutes
Cooking Time: 30 minutes
Serving: 2

Ingredients:

- Bananas, five or six
- Apples, two or three
- Spring onions, three
- Gem lettuce, separated into leaves
- Lime zest, one
- Chili sauce, one teaspoon
- Fish sauce, one tablespoon
- Rice vinegar, one tablespoon
- Sugar, one tablespoon
- Sesame oil, one tablespoon
- Sesame seeds, one cup

Instructions:
1. Take a large bowl to put all the ingredients into it.
2. First of all, slice the bananas into small pieces so that proper mixing can be done.
3. Then slice the apples in the same way.
4. Put them into the bowl.
5. Add chili sauce and fish sauce into the bowl.
6. Add all spices one by one.
7. Add the rice vinegar in such a way equal distribution can be done.
8. Take the gem lettuce in a separate bowl.
9. Add the lime zest and juice into it.
10. Add the spring onions, sesame seeds and sesame oil into it.
11. Mix all the ingredients so that a good paste is formed
12. Then add it in the first bowl with apples and bananas.
13. You can add sugar as per your requirement.
14. Your salad is ready to be served with chili sauce.

5.3 Thai Mung Bean Pudding Recipe

Preparation Time: 10 minutes
Cooking Time: 15 minutes
Serving: 4

Ingredients:
- Tapioca flour, one cup
- Mung beans, half cup
- Coconut milk, half cup
- White sugar, half cup
- Salt, one teaspoon
- Eggs, two
- Lemon extract, one teaspoon
- Almond extract, one teaspoon
- All-purpose flour, two cups
- Butter, one cup

Instructions:
1. Take a medium bowl and add the mung beans in it.
2. Add one cup tapioca flour and mix well.
3. Then refrigerate it.
4. Take a large bowl and add the coconut milk into it.
5. Add the sugar, salt and milk.
6. Mix them well.
7. Mix the warm milk mixture with the flour and the mung beans.
8. Add the eggs, lemon extract and almond extract together.
9. Add the baking soda in the mixture.
10. Simmer it for few minutes.
11. Check the thickness of the pudding.
12. Your dish is ready to be served.

5.4 Thai Mango Sticky Rice Recipe

Preparation Time: 10 minutes
Cooking Time: 10 minutes
Serving: 4

Ingredients:

- Water, one and a half cup
- Ripe mangoes, two
- Thai sweet rice, one cup
- Coconut milk, one can
- Salt, a quarter teaspoon
- Brown sugar, five tablespoon

Instructions:

1. Add half cup of water, rice, plus half can of the coconut milk, the salt, and one tablespoon of the brown sugar.
2. Stir well.
3. Add coconut milk, salt, and some of the brown sugar to the saucepan.
4. Bring to a gentle boil, and then partially cover with a lid.
5. Reduce heat to medium-low, or just until you get a gentle simmer.
6. Simmer thirty minutes, or until the coconut water has been absorbed by the rice.
7. Turn off the heat but leave the pot on the burner with the lid on it tightly.
8. Allow it to stay for five minutes.
9. To make the sauce, warm the remaining coconut milk over medium-low heat.
10. Add three tablespoons of brown sugar, stirring to dissolve.
11. Prepare the mangoes by cutting them open and slicing each into bite-sized pieces.
12. Scoop some warm rice into each serving bowl, and then drizzle lots of the sweet coconut sauce over the top.
13. Arrange mango slices on the rice and finish with a drizzle of more sauce.
14. Your dish is ready to be served.

5.5 Thai Mango Tapioca Pudding Recipe

Preparation Time: 10 minutes

Cooking Time: 10 minutes
Serving: 4

Ingredients:

- Tapioca flour, one cup
- Mangoes, two
- Coconut milk, half cup
- White sugar, half cup
- Salt, one teaspoon
- Eggs, two
- Lemon extract, one teaspoon
- Almond extract, one teaspoon
- All-purpose flour, two cups
- Butter, one cup

Instructions:

1. Take a medium bowl and add the tapioca flour in it.
2. Add the one cup coconut milk and mix well.
3. Then refrigerate it.
4. Take a large bowl and add the spices into it.
5. Add the sugar, salt and mangoes.
6. Mix them well.
7. Mix the warm milk mixture with the flour and the mangoes.
8. Add the eggs, lemon extract and almond extract together.
9. Add the baking soda in the mixture.
10. Simmer it for few minutes.
11. Check the thickness of the pudding.
12. Your dish is ready to be served.

5.6 Thai Fried Bananas Recipe

Preparation Time: 30 minutes
Cooking Time: 10 minutes
Serving: 4

Ingredients:

- Bananas, five

- Cornstarch, one tablespoon
- Water, two cups
- Coconut milk, one cup
- Rice flour, one cup
- Chinese five spice, as needed
- Cooking oil, as required

Instructions:
1. In a large bowl, add all the ingredients together except the bananas and oil.
2. Mix everything to form a consistent mixture.
3. Dip your bananas into the mixture and then fry them in the cooking oil.
4. Fry your bananas until they turn golden brown.
5. Dish out and drizzle maple syrup if you want on top.
6. Your dish is ready to be served.

5.7 Thai Steamed Banana Cake Recipe

Preparation Time: 10 minutes
Cooking Time: 20 minutes
Serving: 4

Ingredients:

- Bananas, five
- Salt, two tablespoon
- White sugar, two cups
- Cornstarch, one tablespoon
- Water, two cups
- Coconut milk, one cup
- Rice flour, one cup
- Pandan essence, as needed
- Raspberries, aa required

Instructions:
1. Take bananas and peel them.
2. Then steam them properly.

3. Take water in a pot and heat it.
4. Take a large bowl and add the sweet rice into it.
5. Cook the rice and add some of sugar into it for taste.
6. Take another bowl and add coconut milk into it.
7. Mix the palm sugar into the coconut milk.
8. Then mix the rice cooked and coconut milk together.
9. Take them into a large bowl after mixing.
10. Add steamed bananas and raspberries into it.
11. Mix them well and then bake your cake.
12. Your cake is ready to be served.

5.8 Thai Tea Cake Recipe

Preparation Time: 10 minutes
Cooking Time: 40 minutes
Serving: 2

Ingredients:

- Tea, one cup
- Salt, two tablespoon
- White sugar, two cups
- Cornstarch, one tablespoon
- Water, two cups
- Coconut milk, one cup
- Rice flour, one cup
- Pandan essence, as needed
- Raspberries, as required

Instructions:

1. Take one cup of tea.
2. Take water in a pot and heat it.
3. Take a large bowl and add the sweet rice into it.
4. Cook the rice and add some of the sugar into it for taste.
5. Take another bowl and add coconut milk into it.
6. Mix the palm sugar into the coconut milk.
7. Then mix the rice cooked and coconut milk together.

8. Take them into a large bowl after mixing.
9. Mix them well and then bake your cake.
10. Your cake is ready to be served.

5.9 Thai Banana Spring Rolls Recipe

Preparation Time: 10 minutes
Cooking Time: 10 minutes
Serving: 2

Ingredients:

- Chopped bananas, five
- Shredded coconut, half cup
- Wonton wraps, as required
- Chinese five spice, as needed
- Cooking oil, as required

Instructions:

1. In a large bowl, mix all the ingredients together.
2. Add the mixture into the wonton wrappers.
3. Wrap your rolls.
4. Fry your rolls until they turn golden brown.
5. Dish out and drizzle any sauce if you want on top.
6. Your dish is ready to be served.

5.10 Thai Mango Cake Recipe

Preparation Time: 30 minutes
Cooking Time: 10 minutes
Serving: 4

Ingredients:

- Mangoes, three
- Salt, two tablespoon
- White sugar, two cups
- Cornstarch, one tablespoon
- Water, two cups
- Coconut milk, one cup
- Rice flour, one cup
- Raspberries, aa required

Instructions:
1. Take the mangoes into a bowl.
2. Slice them into small pieces.
3. Add salt to it for taste as required.
4. Take water in a pot and heat it.
5. Take a large bowl and add the sweet rice into it.
6. Cook the rice and add some of the sugar into it for taste.
7. Take another bowl and add coconut milk into it.
8. Mix the palm sugar into the coconut milk.
9. Then mix the sliced mangoes and coconut milk together.
10. Take them into a large bowl after mixing.
11. Add the coconut juice and raspberries into it.
12. Mix them well.
13. Then bake them for fifteen minutes.
14. After cooking, you can refrigerate the cake.
15. Your cake is ready to be served.

5.11 Thai Coconut Cake Recipe

Preparation Time: 10 minutes
Cooking Time: 10 minutes
Serving: 4

Ingredients:

- Coconut, two
- Salt, two tablespoon
- White sugar, two cups

- Cornstarch, one tablespoon
- Water, two cups
- Coconut milk, one cup
- Rice flour, one cup
- Raspberries, aa required

Instructions:

1. Take the coconut juice into a bowl.
2. Add salt to it for taste as required.
3. Take water in a pot and heat it.
4. Take a large bowl and add the sweet rice into it.
5. Cook the rice and add some of sugar into it for taste.
6. Take another bowl and add coconut milk into it.
7. Mix the palm sugar into the coconut milk.
8. Then mix the rice cooked and coconut milk together.
9. Take them into a large bowl after mixing.
10. Add the coconut juice and raspberries into it.
11. Mix them well.
12. Then bake them for fifteen minutes.
13. After cooking you can refrigerate the cake.
14. Your cake is ready to be served.

5.12 Thai Mango Ice Cream Recipe

Preparation Time: 10 minutes
Cooking Time: 15 minutes
Serving: 2

- Mangoes, two
- Coconut milk, half cup
- White sugar, half cup
- Salt, one teaspoon
- Eggs, two
- Lemon extract, one teaspoon
- Almond extract, one teaspoon
- All-purpose flour, two cups
- Butter, one cup

Instructions:

1. Slice the mangoes into small pieces.
2. Take a medium bowl and add the tapioca flour in it.
3. Add one cup of coconut milk and mix well.
4. Then refrigerate it.
5. Take a large bowl and add the spices into it.
6. Add the sugar, the salt and the spices.
7. Mix them well.
8. Mix the warm milk mixture with the flour and the sliced mangoes.
9. Add the eggs, the lemon extract and the almond extract together.
10. Add the baking soda in the mixture.
11. Simmer it for few minutes.
12. Check the thickness of the ice cream.
13. Refrigerate it.
14. Your dish is ready to be served.

5.13 Thai Sticky Black Rice Pudding Recipe

Preparation Time: 15 minutes
Cooking Time: 25 minutes
Serving: 3

Ingredients:

- Black rice, two cups
- Chinese sweet spices, to taste
- Coconut milk, half cup
- White sugar, half cup
- Salt, one teaspoon
- Eggs, two
- Lemon extract, one teaspoon
- Almond extract, one teaspoon
- All-purpose flour, two cups
- Butter, one cup

Instructions:

1. Cook the black rice in the rice cooking pan.

2. Take a medium bowl and add the tapioca flour in it.
3. Add one cup of coconut milk and mix well.
4. Then refrigerate it.
5. Take a large bowl and add the spices into it.
6. Add the sugar, the salt and the spices.
7. Mix them well.
8. Mix the warm milk mixture with the flour and the cooked rice.
9. Add the eggs, lemon extract and almond extract together.
10. Add the baking soda in the mixture.
11. Simmer it for few minutes.
12. Your dish is ready to be served.

5.14 Thai Egg and Coconut Custard Recipe

Preparation Time: 30 minutes
Cooking Time: 10 minutes
Serving: 4

Ingredients:
- Eggs, two
- Coconut, two
- Chinese sweet spices, to taste
- Coconut milk, half cup
- White sugar, half cup
- Salt, one teaspoon
- Lemon extract, one teaspoon
- Almond extract, one teaspoon
- All-purpose flour, two cups
- Butter, one cup

Instructions:
1. Take a medium bowl and add the eggs and the tapioca flour in it.
2. Add one cup of coconut milk and mix well.
3. Then refrigerate it.
4. Take a large bowl and add the spices into it.
5. Add the sugar, the salt and the beaten eggs.
6. Mix them well.
7. Mix the warm milk mixture with the flour and coconut.

8. Add the eggs, lemon extract and almond extract together.
9. Add the baking soda in the mixture.
10. Simmer it for few minutes.
11. Check the thickness of the custard.
12. Your dish is ready to be served.

5.15 Thai Sweet Corn Pudding Recipe

Preparation Time: 10 minutes
Cooking Time: 30 minutes
Serving: 4

Ingredients:

- Butter, one cup
- Sweet corn, one cup
- Eggs, two
- Cherries, two
- All-purpose flour, two cups
- Water, as required
- Baking soda, one tablespoon
- Salt, a pinch
- Walnuts, one cup

Instructions:
1. Take a large bowl and clean it well.
2. Add the sweet corn and the baking soda.
3. Add the salt and the cream.
4. Mix all the ingredients well.
5. Add beaten eggs into the mixture.
6. Pour into the dish and spread evenly.
7. Take a small bowl and add the sugar and the butter.
8. Mix them until it becomes smooth.
9. Add the mixture into flour and mix well.
10. Simmer it for about twenty-five minutes
11. Your dish is ready to be served.

Chapter 6: The World of Traditional Thai Recipes Eaten Only by Thai People

Following are some classic traditional Thai recipes eaten only by Thai people that are rich in healthy nutrients and you can easily make them with the detailed instructions list given in each recipe:

6.1 Patonga (Thai Breakfast Donut) Recipe

Preparation Time: 15 minutes
Cooking Time: 30 minutes
Serving: 3

Ingredients:

- All-purpose flour, one cup
- Baking soda, one cup
- Sugar, two tablespoon
- Water, half cup
- Vegetable oil, two cups
- Milk, two cups
- Walnuts, one cup
- Eggs, four
- Cherries, one cup
- Butter as needed

Instructions:

1. Take a large bowl and clean it well.
2. Add the sugar and the baking soda.
3. Add the salt and the cream.
4. Mix all the ingredients well.
5. Add beaten eggs into the mixture.
6. Pour into the dish and spread evenly.
7. Take a small bowl and add the sugar and the butter.
8. Mix them until become smooth.
9. Add the mixture into flour and mix well.
10. Bake it for about twenty-five minutes.
11. Your dish is ready to be served.

6. Khanom Kharuk (Thai Mini Pancakes) Recipe

Preparation Time: 30 minutes
Cooking Time: 50 minutes
Serving: 5

Ingredients:

- Blackberry jam, one cup
- Butter, one cup
- Eggs, two
- Cherries, two
- All-purpose flour, two cups
- Water, as required
- Baking soda, one tablespoon
- Salt, a pinch
- Walnuts, one cup

Instructions:
1. Take a large bowl and clean it well.
2. Add the sugar and the baking soda.
3. Add the salt and the cream.
4. Mix all the ingredients well.
5. Add beaten eggs into the mixture.
6. Add blackberry jam into it.
7. Pour into the dish and spread evenly.
8. Take a small bowl and add the sugar and the butter.
9. Mix them until the mixture becomes smooth.
10. Add the mixture into flour and mix well.
11. Bake it for about thirty-five minutes.
12. Your dish is ready to be served.

6.3 Jauk (The Rice Porridge) Recipe

Preparation Time: 20 minutes
Cooking Time: 20 minutes
Serving: 2

Ingredients:

- Fish sauce, three teaspoon
- Brown cooked rice, two cups
- Ground pork, one cup
- Cilantro, one tablespoon
- Black pepper, to taste
- Chicken broth, four cups
- Egg white, half cup
- Galangal, one slice
- Ginger, two tablespoon
- Palm sugar, one tablespoon
- Lime juice, one tablespoon
- Alfa one rice bran oil, teaspoon
- Coconut milk, one cup
- Bean sprouts, one cup
- Fried shallots, to serve
- Red chili, to serve

Instructions:
1. Cook the rice in rice cooker.
2. Then refrigerate it.
3. Prepare meat balls by mixing all the ingredients one by one
4. Cook it for one minute with continuous stirring.
5. Add the coconut milk into the mixture.
6. Boil the coconut milk along with mixture.
7. Continue boiling for five minutes until water reduces to minimum level.
8. Add the egg whites and mix well.
9. Then take the chicken broth in a separate large pot.
10. Add the lemon grass and galangal in it.
11. Simmer it for five minutes.
12. Then add them in already cooked brown rice.
13. Adjust taste by adding pepper and salt.
14. Your soup is ready to be served.
15. Serve it with chilies and soy sauce.

6.4 Khao Tom (The Rice Porridge Soup) Recipe

Preparation Time: 10 minutes
Cooking Time: 25 minutes
Serving: 3

Ingredients:

- Fish sauce, three teaspoon
- Brown cooked rice, two cups
- Ground pork, one cup
- Cilantro, one tablespoon
- Black pepper, to taste
- Chicken broth, four cups
- Egg white, half cup
- Galangal, one slice
- Ginger, two tablespoon
- Palm sugar, one tablespoon
- Lime juice, one tablespoon
- Alfa one rice bran oil, teaspoon
- Coconut milk, one cup
- Bean sprouts, one cup
- Fried shallots, to serve
- Red chili, to serve

Instructions:

1. Cook the rice in rice cooker.
2. Then refrigerate it.
3. Prepare meat balls by mixing all the ingredients one by one
4. Cook it for one minute with continuous stirring.
5. Add the coconut milk into the mixture.
6. Boil the coconut milk along with mixture.
7. Continue boiling for five minutes until water reduces to minimum level.
8. Add the egg white and mix well.
9. Then take the chicken broth in separate large pot.
10. Add the lemon grass and galangal in it.
11. Simmer it for five minutes.
12. Then add them in already cooked brown rice.
13. Adjust taste by adding pepper and salt.
14. Your soup is ready to be served.
15. Serve it with chilies and soy sauce.

6.5 Dim Sum (Thai Steamed Buns) Recipe

Preparation Time: 50 minutes

Cooking Time: 30 minutes
Serving: 4

Ingredients:

- Ground pork, half pound
- Thin soy sauce, one tablespoon
- Thai pepper powder, half tablespoon
- Sugar, one tablespoon
- Garlic powder, one tablespoon
- Fresh shallot, half tablespoon
- Milk, one cup
- Vegetable oil, one tablespoon
- All-purpose flour, one cup
- Whole wheat flour, half cup
- Salt, to taste
- Water, to kneed
- Cucumber, one
- Yeast, one cup

Instructions:
1. Take a bowl and add the flour into it.
2. Then add the yeast and sugar into it.
3. Add lukewarm water in it.
4. Set aside for half an hour.
5. In another bowl, take the whole wheat flour.
6. Add the yeast dough in it.
7. Then add the salt and some water in it.
8. Then combine the ingredients to form a soft dough.
9. Kneed it for ten minutes.
10. Meanwhile, chop all the vegetables.
11. Mix them with soy sauce, chili vinegar, sugar and salt.
12. Make round forms of dough with the help of the oil.
13. Then bake your buns for ten minutes.
14. Once the buns are steamed, take them out.
15. You can serve Thai buns with salad.

6.6 Thai Sweet Rice Cakes Recipe

Preparation Time: 2 minutes

Cooking Time: 25 minutes
Serving: 2

Ingredients:

- Thai sweet rice, two cups
- Salt, two tablespoon
- White sugar, two cups
- Cornstarch, one tablespoon
- Water, two cups
- Coconut milk, one cup
- Rice flour, one cup
- Pandan essence, as needed
- Raspberries, aa required

Instructions:

1. Take a blender and blend the pandan leaves.
2. Then add the paste type material into a bowl.
3. Press the paste so that all juice comes out.
4. Take the juice and discard the solids.
5. Take water in a pot and heat it.
6. Take a large bowl and add the sweet rice into it.
7. Cook the rice and add some of the sugar into it for taste.
8. Take another bowl and add coconut milk into it.
9. Mix the palm sugar into the coconut milk.
10. Then mix the cooked rice and coconut milk together.
11. Take them into a large bowl after mixing.
12. Add pandan juice and raspberries into it.
13. Mix them well.
14. Then bake them well.
15. After cooking you can refrigerate the cake.
16. Your cake is ready to be served.

6.7 Thai Steamed Pandan Cakes Recipe

Preparation Time: 15 minutes
Cooking Time: 35 minutes
Serving: 2

Ingredients:

- Pandan leaves, one bunch
- Tapioca starch, one cup
- Arrowroot starch, one cup
- Water, two cups
- Coconut milk, one cup
- Rice flour, one cup
- Jasmine tea, one cup

Instructions:
1. Take a blender and blend the pandan leaves.
2. Then add the paste type material into a bowl.
3. Press the paste so that all juice comes out.
4. Take the juice and discard the solids.
5. Take water in a pot and heat it.
6. Take a large bowl and add rice flour into it.
7. Then whisk it with tapioca starch and arrowroot starch.
8. Take another bowl and add coconut milk into it.
9. Mix the palm sugar into the coconut milk.
10. Then mix the rice flour and coconut milk together.
11. Take them into a large bowl after mixing.
12. Add pandan juice and jasmine tea into it.
13. Mix them well and cook them efficiently.
14. After cooking you can refrigerate the whole food.
15. Your cake is ready to be served.

6.8 Thai Carrot and Radish Salad Recipe

Preparation Time: 5 minutes
Cooking Time: 5 minutes
Serving: 3

Ingredients:

- Carrots, two
- Radishes, ten
- Spring onions, three
- Gem lettuce, separated into leaves

- Lime zest, one
- Chili sauce, one teaspoon
- Fish sauce, one tablespoon
- Rice vinegar, one tablespoon
- Sugar, one tablespoon
- Sesame oil, one tablespoon
- Sesame seeds, one cup

Instructions:

1. Take a large bowl to put all the ingredients into it.
2. First of all, slice the carrots into small pieces so that proper mixing can be done.
3. Then slice the radish in the same way.
4. Put them into the bowl.
5. Add chili sauce and fish sauce into the bowl.
6. Add all spices one by one.
7. Add the rice vinegar in such a way that equal distribution can be done.
8. Take the gem lettuce in a separate bowl.
9. Add the lime zest and juice into it.
10. Add the spring onions, sesame seeds and sesame oil into it.
11. Mix all the ingredients so that a good paste is formed
12. Then add it in the first bowl with carrots and radishes.
13. You can add sugar as per your requirement.
14. Your salad is ready to be served with chili sauce.

6.9 Thai Fish Broth with Vegetables Recipe

Preparation Time: 10 minutes
Cooking Time: 25 minutes
Serving: 4

Ingredients:

- Brown rice noodles, one cup
- Chicken, two cups
- Red curry paste, one teaspoon
- Fish sauce, one tablespoon
- White fish, one bowl
- Red chili, to serve
- Prawns, one cup

- Fried shallots, to serve
- Salt, to taste
- Pepper, to taste
- Lime leaves, one cup

Instructions:

1. Take a large saucepan and add oil in it.
2. Heat it over medium high heat.
3. Add the brown rice noodles into it.
4. Cook it for one minute with the continuous stirring.
5. Add the chicken into the mixture.
6. Boil the chicken and curry paste along with mixture.
7. Continue boiling for five minutes until water reduces to minimum level.
8. Add the lime leaves in a separate bowl.
9. And cover it with the boiling water for five minutes.
10. Add fish into the mixture and boil until the meat becomes soft and tender.
11. Add the fish sauce, lime juice and peas into the mixture.
12. Add the prawns to the mixture in the end having all the ingredients.
13. Cook for five minutes so that color and texture of the fish become suitable.
14. Your dish is ready to be served with the sauces and spices you want.

6.10 Thai Prawn and Coconut Soup Recipe

Preparation Time: 10 minutes
Cooking Time: 25 minutes
Serving: 2

Ingredients:

- sauce, three teaspoon
- Palm sugar, one tablespoon
- Lime juice, one tablespoon
- Peas, trimmed, one cup
- Peeled prawns, two cups
- Alfa one rice bran oil, teaspoon
- Coconut milk, one cup
- Bean sprouts, one cup
- Fried shallots, to serve
- Red chili, to serve
- Red curry paste, half cup

- Noodles, one packet

Instructions:

1. Take a large saucepan and add oil in it.
2. Heat it over medium high heat.
3. Add curry paste into it.
4. Cook it for one minute with continuous stirring.
5. Add the coconut milk into the mixture.
6. Boil the coconut milk along with mixture.
7. Continue boiling for five minutes until water reduces to minimum level.
8. Add the noodles in a separate bowl.
9. Cover it with the boiling water for five minutes.
10. Then remove the noodles with the help of fork and drain it.
11. Add the fish sauce, lime juice and peas into the mixture.
12. Add the prawns to the soup.
13. Cook for five minutes.
14. Your soup is ready to be served.

Conclusion

While living a busy life, food becomes the one of the source of happiness for individuals in the 21st century. Different cuisines are available in the world and each of them being totally different from the other, adds delight to the people's lives. Thai cuisine covers dishes from Thailand and Thai foods which are extremely popular in the whole world.

In this book, we have discussed different aspects of Thai cuisine and not only the recipes. We discussed in detail the history and origin of Thai foods. The various spices used in Thai cooking have enormous amount of amazing properties that has such positive and healthy impact on our overall health. This cookbook includes 70 recipes that consist of breakfast, lunch, dinner, dessert, and the recipes that are only eaten by Thai people. You can easily make these recipes at home without supervision of any kind. So start cooking today and enjoy the Thai cuisine more than ever.